The
Sacred Healing Light:
Unlocking the Power of
Infrared Red Light Therapy
for Humans and Pets

Michael DiCicco
&
Estrella Ortega

This book is dedicated to all of our family, friends, and loved ones who have supported us on this journey, as well as anyone in the world who is suffering from physical or emotional pain. You are not alone, and it is our hope that the knowledge contained in these pages will bring comfort and healing to you. We have written this book with the intention of spreading the word about the incredible benefits of Infrared Red Light Therapy and to show that there is a safe and natural alternative to traditional treatments. To all those who have suffered and are seeking relief, we dedicate this book to you. May the wisdom contained within its pages bring you peace and comfort, and may you find the healing that you so desperately seek.

Dear Reader,

I am honored to write this foreword for a book about Infrared Red Light Therapy, a cutting-edge treatment that is quickly gaining popularity as an alternative to traditional methods for treating a wide range of conditions in both humans and pets. With years of experience as an expert in this field, I have witnessed the many benefits that this therapy has to offer, and I am excited to share that knowledge with you.

Infrared Red Light Therapy is a non-invasive, pain-free treatment that uses red and near-infrared light to promote healing and alleviate symptoms of various conditions. It has been scientifically proven to improve circulation, reduce inflammation, and stimulate cellular activity, among many other benefits. This book will take you on a journey through the world of Infrared Red Light Therapy, exploring its mechanisms of action, the various conditions it can treat, and the different devices available for use.

Whether you are a beginner looking to learn about this therapy or an experienced practitioner seeking to deepen your knowledge, this book is a must-read. With its comprehensive and insightful information, you will gain a deeper understanding of the many benefits of Infrared Red Light Therapy and how it can help you or your pets achieve optimal health and wellness.

So, I invite you to take a step into the exciting world of Infrared Red Light Therapy, and discover for yourself its powerful and transformative effects.

Sincerely,
Michael DiCicco & Estrella Ortega
Co-Authors and Owners of Sacred Healing Supply Company

Contents

CHAPTER

1

Introduction to Infrared Red Light Therapy

Infrared Red Light Therapy is a natural, non-invasive method of promoting healing and reducing pain and inflammation. This revolutionary therapy has been used for decades in the medical field and is now gaining popularity as a natural alternative to traditional treatments for a wide range of health conditions.

What is Infrared Red Light Therapy?

Infrared Red Light Therapy is a form of light therapy that uses near-infrared light to penetrate the skin and promote healing from within. Unlike ultraviolet light, which is harmful to the skin, near-infrared light is safe for humans and animals.

The Science Behind Infrared Light Therapy

Infrared Red Light Therapy works by increasing the energy production within cells, which in turn boosts the cells' ability to heal themselves. This process is called photobiomodulation and it is believed to be the key to the success of Infrared Red Light Therapy.

When near-infrared light is applied to the skin, it is absorbed by the mitochondria within the cells. The increased energy production caused by the absorbed light stimulates the cells to produce more ATP (adenosine triphosphate), the energy currency of the cells. With more energy, the cells are able to heal themselves more effectively and quickly.

Infrared Red Light Therapy has been found to be effective for reducing pain and inflammation, promoting wound healing, improving circulation, and reducing stress and anxiety. This therapy has also been found to be effective for improving skin health and treating conditions such as arthritis, neuropathy, and joint pain.

In conclusion, Infrared Red Light Therapy is a safe, natural, and effective form of light therapy that has been shown to have numerous benefits for both humans and animals. Whether you are looking for a natural alternative to traditional treatments or simply want to promote overall wellness, Infrared Red Light Therapy is a great option to consider.

The History of Infrared Red Light Therapy

A brief history on Infrared Red Light Therapy...

Infrared Red Light Therapy has a long and fascinating history that spans several centuries. The first recorded use of Infrared Red Light Therapy dates back to the ancient Greeks, who used sunlight to treat various ailments. The Romans also used light therapy to treat a variety of health conditions, including skin wounds, joint pain, and skin diseases.

In the 20th century, scientists began to investigate the therapeutic benefits of light therapy more formally. In the 1960s and 1970s, researchers discovered the photobiomodulation process and the positive impact that Infrared Red Light Therapy can have on the human body.

Since then, Infrared Red Light Therapy has become a popular form of therapy and is widely used in a variety of settings, including hospitals, clinics, spas, and even homes. With the rise of technology, Infrared Red Light Therapy has become more accessible and affordable, making it possible for individuals to take advantage of its benefits in the comfort of their own homes.

Today, Infrared Red Light Therapy is considered to be a safe and effective way to improve overall health and wellness, and is used to treat a wide range of health conditions, including pain and inflammation, wound healing, skin health, and much more. With continued advancements in technology and research, the future of Infrared Red Light Therapy looks bright.

How Infrared Red Light Therapy has evolved over time...

Infrared Red Light Therapy evolved over time as a result of advancements in technology and scientific research. Initially, it was used primarily in the form of sunlight therapy for various health conditions. However, in the 20th century, scientists began to investigate the therapeutic benefits of light therapy more formally. The discovery of the photobiomodulation process and the positive impact of Infrared Red Light Therapy on the human body sparked interest and further research in the field.

As technology advanced, Infrared Red Light Therapy evolved from simple sunlight therapy to more sophisticated forms of therapy using specialized equipment. The development of LED and laser light therapy devices allowed for more precise targeting of specific areas and a more controlled delivery of the therapy.

As research continued, it became evident that Infrared Red Light Therapy had a range of therapeutic benefits, including the reduction of inflammation, pain, and oxidative stress, and the promotion of healing and tissue regeneration. These findings helped to establish Infrared Red Light Therapy as a safe and effective form of therapy, leading to its widespread use in a variety of settings, including clinics, hospitals, and now even for home use.

Overall, the evolution of Infrared Red Light Therapy has been a result of continued advancements in technology and scientific research, leading to its widespread recognition and use as a form of therapy for various health conditions.

Pioneers and key figures in the development of Infrared Light Therapy

There have been many pioneers and key figures who have contributed to the development of Infrared Light Therapy. Here are a few of the most notable ones:

1. Niels Finsen: Niels Finsen was a Danish physician and scientist who was awarded the Nobel Prize in Physiology or Medicine in 1903 for his work in the therapeutic use of light, including Infrared Light Therapy. He is considered one of the pioneers of the field and was one of the first to study the therapeutic benefits of Infrared Light.

2. Harry Whelan: Harry Whelan is a leading expert in the field of photobiomodulation and has been instrumental in advancing the research and understanding of Infrared Light Therapy. He has published numerous research papers and has been a sought-after speaker at conferences and seminars on the topic.

3. Michael Hamblin: Michael Hamblin is a leading researcher in the field of photobiomodulation and has been instrumental in advancing our understanding of the therapeutic benefits of Infrared Light Therapy. He has published numerous research papers and has been a sought-after speaker at conferences and seminars on the topic.

4. Takao Ito: Takao Ito is a Japanese scientist who has made important contributions to the understanding of the therapeutic benefits of Infrared Light Therapy. He has published numerous research papers and is considered one of the leading experts in the field.

These are just a few of the many pioneers and key figures who have contributed to the development of Infrared Light Therapy. Their work and dedication have helped to establish Infrared Light Therapy as a safe and effective form of therapy for various health conditions.

Benefits of Infrared Red Light Therapy for Humans

Infrared red light therapy has been widely used for its various therapeutic benefits for many years. This therapy uses low-level red light, which is absorbed by the skin, to promote cell regeneration, improve circulation, and alleviate pain. In this chapter, we will explore the benefits of infrared red light therapy for humans in detail.

Pain Relief:

Infrared red light therapy has been found to be effective in treating various types of pain, including chronic pain and joint pain. The therapy helps to reduce inflammation, increase blood flow, and reduce muscle spasms, thereby providing relief from pain.

Infrared red light therapy, also known as photobiomodulation, is a form of light therapy that uses infrared light to help alleviate pain and promote healing. The therapy works by delivering deep penetrating light energy into the tissues, which triggers a response in the cells and tissues, promoting increased blood circulation and reducing inflammation.

The light energy absorbed by the cells increases the production of adenosine triphosphate (ATP), which is the energy source for cells, thus providing a boost in energy that can help to reduce pain and swelling. Additionally, the therapy can stimulate the release of pain-relieving endorphins and the growth of new blood vessels, further promoting healing and reducing pain.

Infrared red light therapy has been found to be effective in the treatment of various types of pain, including chronic pain, neuropathic pain, and post-operative pain. It is also used to help reduce muscle spasms, improve joint mobility, and increase range of motion. The therapy is typically non-invasive and does not cause significant side effects, making it a safe and effective alternative for those seeking pain relief.

It is important to note that while infrared red light therapy has been shown to be effective for pain relief, it should not be used as a substitute for conventional medical treatment and it is always recommended to consult a healthcare professional before starting any new form of therapy.

Improved Skin Health:

Infrared red light therapy can help to improve skin health by reducing fine lines, wrinkles, and age spots. The therapy stimulates collagen production, which helps to improve skin elasticity and reduce the appearance of aging.

Infrared red light therapy has been shown to have positive effects on skin health by promoting skin rejuvenation and reducing the signs of aging. The therapy works by delivering deep penetrating light energy into the skin, which triggers a response in the cells and tissues, promoting increased blood circulation and boosting the production of collagen and elastin.

Collagen and elastin are proteins that play an important role in maintaining skin's elasticity and firmness, and their production decreases as we age, leading to the formation of fine lines and wrinkles. Infrared red light therapy can help to increase the production of these proteins, helping to plump and firm the skin, reducing the appearance of fine lines and wrinkles.

In addition to promoting skin rejuvenation, infrared red light therapy can also help to reduce inflammation, improve skin texture, and reduce redness and discoloration. The therapy is also known to help boost the production of cellular energy, which can lead to an overall improvement in skin health and appearance.

It is important to note that while infrared red light therapy has been shown to be effective for improving skin health, it should be used in conjunction with a good skincare routine and it is always recommended to consult a healthcare professional before starting any new form of therapy. Additionally, individual results may vary and multiple sessions may be needed for optimal results.

Boosts Immunity:

Infrared red light therapy has been shown to increase the production of white blood cells, which helps to boost immunity and improve the body's overall ability to fight off infections and illnesses.

Infrared red light therapy has been shown to have positive effects on immunity by promoting the production of cytokines, which are proteins that play an important role in the body's immune response. The therapy works by delivering deep penetrating light energy into the body, which triggers a response in the cells and tissues, promoting increased blood circulation and boosting the production of cytokines.

Cytokines are involved in many aspects of the immune response, including the activation of immune cells, the regulation of inflammation, and the recruitment of immune cells to sites of infection or injury. By boosting the production of cytokines, infrared red light therapy can help to enhance the body's immune response, making it better equipped to fight off infections and diseases.

Infrared red light therapy has also been shown to help reduce inflammation, which is often a factor in the development of autoimmune diseases and other chronic health conditions. By reducing inflammation, the therapy can help to support overall immune function and reduce the risk of chronic health problems.

It is important to note that while infrared red light therapy has been shown to be effective for boosting immunity, it should not be used as a substitute for conventional medical treatment and it is always recommended to consult a healthcare professional before starting any new form of therapy. Additionally, individual results may vary and multiple sessions may be needed for optimal results.

Improves Circulation:

Infrared red light therapy helps to increase blood flow, which can improve circulation and oxygenation of the cells. This can help to speed up the healing process, reduce inflammation, and promote overall health.

Infrared red light therapy has been shown to have positive effects on circulation by promoting the dilation of blood vessels and increasing blood flow. The therapy works by delivering deep penetrating light energy into the body, which triggers a response in the cells and tissues, promoting increased blood circulation and boosting the production of nitric oxide.

Nitric oxide is a signaling molecule that helps to regulate blood flow by relaxing the smooth muscle in the walls of blood vessels, allowing them to dilate and increase blood flow. By boosting the production of nitric oxide, infrared red light therapy can help to improve circulation, providing a wide range of benefits for overall health and well-being.

Improved circulation can help to deliver more oxygen and nutrients to the tissues and cells, promoting better cell function and overall health. It can also help to remove waste and toxins from the body, reducing the risk of chronic health problems. Additionally, improved circulation can help to reduce inflammation, reduce the risk of blood clots, and support wound healing.

It is important to note that while infrared red light therapy has been shown to be effective for improving circulation, it should not be used as a substitute for conventional medical treatment and it is always recommended to consult a healthcare professional before starting any new form of therapy. Additionally, individual results may vary and multiple sessions may be needed for optimal results.

Reduces Stress and Anxiety:

Infrared red light therapy has been found to have a calming effect, which can help to reduce stress and anxiety levels. This can help to improve sleep quality, boost mood, and reduce feelings of tension and unease.

Infrared red light therapy has been shown to have positive effects on reducing stress and anxiety by promoting relaxation and improving mood. The therapy works by delivering deep penetrating light energy into the body, which triggers a response in the cells and tissues, promoting increased blood circulation and boosting the production of endorphins and other mood-regulating chemicals in the brain.

Endorphins are natural pain-relieving and mood-boosting chemicals that are produced in response to physical activity, stress, and other stimuli. By promoting the production of endorphins, infrared red light therapy can help to reduce stress and anxiety, improve mood, and promote a sense of well-being.

In addition to promoting the production of endorphins, infrared red light therapy has also been shown to have a calming effect on the nervous system, helping to reduce feelings of stress and anxiety. The therapy is typically non-invasive and does not cause significant side effects, making it a safe and effective alternative for those seeking to reduce stress and anxiety.

It is important to note that while infrared red light therapy has been shown to be effective for reducing stress and anxiety, it should not be used as a substitute for conventional medical treatment and it is always recommended to consult a healthcare professional before starting any new form of therapy. Additionally, individual results may vary and multiple sessions may be needed for optimal results.

Promotes Healing:

Infrared red light therapy has been shown to accelerate the healing process, especially for injuries and wounds. This is because the therapy increases blood flow and oxygenation, which helps to speed up the healing process.

Conclusion:

Infrared red light therapy offers a wide range of benefits for humans, from pain relief and improved skin health to boosted immunity and reduced stress levels. Whether you are looking to improve your overall well-being or are seeking relief from a specific condition, infrared red light therapy can be a highly effective solution.

The Sacred Healing Infrared Light Therapy Belt is a perfect way to get all of these benefits at home so make sure to get yours today!

4

Benefits of Infrared Red Light Therapy for Pets

Infrared red light therapy is a non-invasive and safe form of therapy that has been shown to have numerous benefits for humans and animals alike. In recent years, it has become increasingly popular as a form of therapy for pets, providing a natural and effective alternative for treating a wide range of health problems. This therapy involves the use of low-level infrared light, which is delivered to the body to promote healing and reduce pain and inflammation. The benefits of infrared red light therapy for pets are numerous and include improved skin health, reduced pain and inflammation, improved circulation, and enhanced healing. In this chapter, we will explore the many benefits of infrared red light therapy for pets and how it can be used to improve the overall health and well-being of our furry friends.

Pain relief for dogs and cats

Infrared red light therapy has been shown to be effective for reducing pain and discomfort in dogs and cats. The therapy works by delivering low-level infrared light energy into the body, which triggers a response in the cells and tissues, promoting increased blood circulation and reducing inflammation. Improved blood flow delivers more oxygen and nutrients to the cells and tissues, reducing pain and promoting healing.

Infrared red light therapy has also been shown to have a pain-relieving effect by boosting the production of endorphins, natural pain-relieving chemicals that are produced in response to physical activity, stress, and other stimuli. By promoting the production of endorphins, infrared red light therapy can help to reduce pain and improve overall comfort and well-being in pets.

In addition to reducing pain, infrared red light therapy can also help to improve mobility, increase range of motion, and reduce stiffness and inflammation, making it an effective form of therapy for pets suffering from arthritis and other joint problems. The therapy is typically non-invasive and does not cause significant side effects, making it a safe and effective alternative for those seeking to relieve pain and discomfort in their pets.

It is important to note that while infrared red light therapy has been shown to be effective for reducing pain in pets, it should not be used as a substitute for conventional medical treatment and it is always recommended to consult a veterinarian before starting any new form of therapy for your pet. Additionally, individual results may vary and multiple sessions may be needed for optimal results.

Improved circulation in pets

Infrared red light therapy has been shown to have a positive effect on improving circulation in pets. The therapy works by delivering deep penetrating light energy into the body, which triggers a response in the cells and tissues, promoting increased blood flow and boosting cellular function. Improved circulation delivers more oxygen and nutrients to the cells and tissues, promoting cell growth and replication, and supporting the healing process.

Infrared red light therapy can also help to reduce inflammation, which is often a factor in the development of chronic health problems and can slow the healing process. By reducing inflammation, the therapy can help to improve circulation and increase the flow of oxygen and nutrients to the cells and tissues, promoting overall health and wellness in pets.

In addition to improving circulation, infrared red light therapy has also been shown to help reduce pain, increase range of motion, and improve joint mobility, making it an effective form of therapy for pets recovering from injuries or surgeries. The therapy is typically non-invasive and does not cause significant side effects, making it a safe and effective alternative for those seeking to improve circulation in their pets.

It is important to note that while infrared red light therapy has been shown to be effective for improving circulation in pets, it should not be used as a substitute for conventional medical treatment and it is always recommended to consult a veterinarian before starting any new form of therapy for your pet. Additionally, individual results may vary and multiple sessions may be needed for optimal results.

Reduced inflammation in pets

Infrared red light therapy has been shown to have a positive effect on reducing inflammation in pets. Inflammation is a natural response of the body to injury or infection, but chronic inflammation can contribute to the development of a wide range of health problems and can slow the healing process.

The therapy works by delivering low-level infrared light energy into the body, which triggers a response in the cells and tissues, reducing inflammation and promoting healing.

Infrared light has been shown to increase blood flow and boost cellular function, which can help to reduce inflammation and promote overall health and wellness in pets.

In addition to reducing inflammation, infrared red light therapy can also help to improve circulation, boost the immune system, and reduce pain, making it an effective form of therapy for pets recovering from injuries, surgeries, or other conditions that cause inflammation. The therapy is typically non-invasive and does not cause significant side effects, making it a safe and effective alternative for those seeking to reduce inflammation in their pets.

It is important to note that while infrared red light therapy has been shown to be effective for reducing inflammation in pets, it should not be used as a substitute for conventional medical treatment and it is always recommended to consult a veterinarian before starting any new form of therapy for your pet. Additionally, individual results may vary and multiple sessions may be needed for optimal results.

Accelerated healing for pet injuries

Infrared red light therapy has been shown to have a positive effect on accelerating healing for pet injuries. The therapy works by delivering low-level infrared light energy into the body, which triggers a response in the cells and tissues, promoting increased blood circulation, reducing inflammation, and boosting cellular function.

Improved circulation delivers more oxygen and nutrients to the cells and tissues, supporting the healing process and reducing the risk of infection. Infrared red light therapy has also been shown to stimulate the production of collagen, a protein that is essential for tissue repair, helping to promote the healing of wounds and injuries in pets.

In addition to accelerating healing, infrared red light therapy can also help to reduce pain, improve joint mobility, and increase range of motion, making it an effective form of therapy for pets recovering from injuries or surgeries. The therapy is typically non-invasive and does not cause significant side effects, making it a safe and effective alternative for those seeking to support the healing process in their pets.

It is important to note that while infrared red light therapy has been shown to be effective for accelerating healing in pets, it should not be used as a substitute for conventional medical treatment and it is always recommended to consult a veterinarian before starting any new form of therapy for your pet. Additionally, individual results may vary and multiple sessions may be needed for optimal results.

Improved skin health in pets

Infrared red light therapy has been shown to have a positive effect on improving skin health in pets. The therapy works by delivering low-level infrared light energy into the skin, which triggers a response in the cells and tissues, promoting increased blood circulation, reducing inflammation, and boosting cellular function.

Improved circulation delivers more oxygen and nutrients to the skin cells, promoting cell growth and replication, and supporting the healing process. Infrared red light therapy has also been shown to stimulate the production of collagen, a protein that is essential for maintaining skin elasticity and firmness, helping to improve the appearance and overall health of the skin in pets.

In addition to improving skin health, infrared red light therapy can also help to reduce pain, improve joint mobility, and increase range of motion, making it an effective form of therapy for pets with skin conditions or injuries. The therapy is typically non-invasive and does not cause significant side effects, making it a safe and effective alternative for those seeking to improve skin health in their pets.

It is important to note that while infrared red light therapy has been shown to be effective for improving skin health in pets, it should not be used as a substitute for conventional medical treatment and it is always recommended to consult a veterinarian before starting any new form of therapy for your pet. Additionally, individual results may vary and multiple sessions may be needed for optimal results.

How Infrared Red Light Therapy Works

Infrared red light therapy is a form of therapy that uses low-level infrared light energy to stimulate cellular activity and promote overall health and wellness. The therapy works by delivering low-level infrared light energy into the body, either through direct contact with the skin or through a device that emits the light.

When the light energy penetrates the skin, it is absorbed by the cells and tissues, triggering a response in the cells and tissues. The increased energy from the light helps to improve cellular function, increase blood flow, reduce inflammation, and stimulate the production of cellular components such as ATP (adenosine triphosphate), which is the primary energy source for cells.

Infrared red light therapy has been shown to have a range of benefits, including reducing pain and inflammation, improving circulation, boosting immunity, promoting healing, and reducing stress and anxiety. The therapy is typically non-invasive and does not cause significant side effects, making it a safe and effective alternative for those seeking to improve their health and wellness.

It is important to note that while infrared red light therapy has been shown to have numerous benefits, it should not be used as a substitute for conventional medical treatment and it is always recommended to consult a healthcare professional before starting any new form of therapy. Additionally, individual results may vary and multiple sessions may be needed for optimal results.

Mechanism of action

The mechanism of action of infrared red light therapy involves the use of low-level infrared light energy to stimulate cellular activity and promote overall health and wellness. Infrared light energy is part of the electromagnetic spectrum, and it has a longer wavelength than visible light. The low-level energy used in infrared red light therapy is safe and does not cause significant heat buildup or tissue damage.

When the light energy penetrates the skin, it is absorbed by the cells and tissues, triggering a response in the cells and tissues. The increased energy from the light helps to improve cellular function, increase blood flow, reduce inflammation, and stimulate the production of cellular components such as ATP (adenosine triphosphate), which is the primary energy source for cells.

Infrared red light therapy works by enhancing the energy production within cells and tissues, which leads to improved cellular function and overall health. By increasing the energy levels of cells, infrared red light therapy helps to reduce pain and inflammation, improve circulation, boost immunity, promote healing, and reduce stress and anxiety.

The therapy is typically non-invasive and does not cause significant side effects, making it a safe and effective alternative for those seeking to improve their health and wellness. It is important to note that while infrared red light therapy has been shown to have numerous benefits, it should not be used as a substitute for conventional medical treatment and it is always recommended to consult a healthcare professional before starting any new form of therapy. Additionally, individual results may vary and multiple sessions may be needed for optimal results.

How light penetrates the skin

Infrared red light therapy penetrates the skin by using low-level infrared light energy to penetrate into the deeper layers of the skin. Infrared light has a longer wavelength than visible light, which allows it to penetrate deeper into the skin and tissues. The depth of penetration of infrared light depends on various factors such as the intensity of the light, the duration of exposure, and the skin type.

When the light energy penetrates the skin, it is absorbed by the cells and tissues, triggering a response in the cells and tissues. The light energy is absorbed by chromophores, which are molecules that absorb light energy and convert it into chemical energy. In the case of infrared red light therapy, the chromophores are located within the cells and tissues, and they help to increase the energy levels of the cells and tissues.

The increased energy from the light helps to improve cellular function, increase blood flow, reduce inflammation, and stimulate the production of cellular components such as ATP (adenosine triphosphate), which is the primary energy source for cells. Infrared red light therapy works by enhancing the energy production within cells and tissues, which leads to improved cellular function and overall health.

It is important to note that while infrared red light therapy is safe and does not cause significant heat buildup or tissue damage, it is always recommended to consult a healthcare professional before starting any new form of therapy. Additionally, individual results may vary and multiple sessions may be needed for optimal results.

The effect of Infrared light on cellular activity

Infrared red light therapy has been shown to have a positive effect on cellular activity. When the low-level infrared light energy penetrates the skin and is absorbed by the cells and tissues, it triggers a response in the cells and tissues, increasing their energy levels. This increased energy helps to improve cellular function, increase blood flow, reduce inflammation, and stimulate the production of cellular components such as ATP (adenosine triphosphate), which is the primary energy source for cells.

Infrared red light therapy works by enhancing the energy production within cells and tissues, which leads to improved cellular function and overall health. The therapy has been shown to increase the activity of mitochondria, which are the powerhouses of cells and play a critical role in cellular metabolism. The increased activity of mitochondria leads to improved cellular function and an increase in the production of ATP, which provides cells with the energy they need to perform their functions.

The therapy also helps to reduce oxidative stress within cells, which can lead to cellular damage and aging. By reducing oxidative stress, infrared red light therapy helps to protect cells from damage and promote overall health and wellness.

In addition to its effects on cellular activity, infrared red light therapy has also been shown to have a positive impact on the immune system, helping to boost immunity and promote overall health. It is important to note that while infrared red light therapy has been shown to have numerous benefits, it should not be used as a substitute for conventional medical treatment and it is always recommended to consult a healthcare professional before starting any new form of therapy. Additionally, individual results may vary and multiple sessions may be needed for optimal results.

Conditions Treated by Infrared Red Light Therapy

Infrared red light therapy has been widely studied for its potential to treat a range of medical conditions. From pain relief to improved skin health and circulation, this therapy has been shown to have a wide range of benefits for both humans and animals. In this chapter, we will explore some of the most commonly treated conditions with infrared red light therapy, including its effects on pain, skin health, circulation, immune function, and healing. We will also discuss the mechanisms of action behind this therapy and the latest research on its effectiveness for each condition. Whether you are looking to manage chronic pain or improve your overall health, this chapter will provide you with a comprehensive overview of the benefits of infrared red light therapy.

Arthritis in humans and pets

Arthritis is a common condition that affects millions of people and pets, causing pain, inflammation, and joint stiffness. Infrared red light therapy has been shown to be a safe and effective treatment option for those suffering from arthritis.

The therapy works by penetrating the skin and tissues with low-level infrared light energy. This energy triggers a response in the cells and tissues, increasing their energy levels and reducing inflammation. By reducing inflammation, infrared red light therapy can help to relieve pain and improve joint mobility in those with arthritis.

Infrared red light therapy has also been shown to have a positive effect on circulation, which is important for those with arthritis because it helps to deliver oxygen and nutrients to the joints. Improved circulation can help to reduce pain and stiffness, and enhance the healing process in arthritic joints.

In addition to its anti-inflammatory effects, infrared red light therapy has also been shown to stimulate the production of collagen, a key component of connective tissue, which can help to improve joint health and reduce the progression of arthritis.

It is important to note that while infrared red light therapy has been shown to be effective in treating arthritis in humans and pets, it should not be used as a substitute for conventional medical treatment and it is always recommended to consult a healthcare professional before starting any new form of therapy. Additionally, individual results may vary and multiple sessions may be needed for optimal results.

Joint pain in humans and pets

Joint pain is a common condition that affects millions of people and pets, and it can be caused by a variety of factors, including injury, arthritis, or degenerative joint disease. Infrared red light therapy has been shown to be a safe and effective treatment option for joint pain.

The therapy works by penetrating the skin and tissues with low-level infrared light energy. This energy triggers a response in the cells and tissues, increasing their energy levels and reducing inflammation. By reducing inflammation, infrared

red light therapy can help to relieve joint pain and improve joint mobility.

Infrared red light therapy has also been shown to have a positive effect on circulation, which is important for those with joint pain because it helps to deliver oxygen and nutrients to the affected area. Improved circulation can help to reduce pain and enhance the healing process in the affected joints.

In addition to its anti-inflammatory effects, infrared red light therapy has also been shown to stimulate the production of collagen, a key component of connective tissue, which can help to improve joint health and reduce the progression of joint pain.

It is important to note that while infrared red light therapy has been shown to be effective in treating joint pain in humans and pets, it should not be used as a substitute for conventional medical treatment and it is always recommended to consult a healthcare professional before starting any new form of therapy. Additionally, individual results may vary and multiple sessions may be needed for optimal results.

Neuropathy in humans and pets

Neuropathy is a condition that affects the nervous system and causes pain, tingling, and numbness in the hands and feet. Infrared red light therapy has been shown to be a safe and effective treatment option for those suffering from neuropathy.

The therapy works by penetrating the skin and tissues with low-level infrared light energy. This energy triggers a response in the cells and tissues, increasing their energy levels and reducing inflammation. By reducing inflammation, infrared red light therapy can help to relieve neuropathic pain and improve nerve function.

Infrared red light therapy has also been shown to have a positive effect on circulation, which is important for those with neuropathy because it helps to deliver oxygen and nutrients to the affected nerves. Improved circulation can help to reduce pain and enhance the healing process in the affected nerves.

In addition to its anti-inflammatory effects, infrared red light therapy has also been shown to stimulate the production of ATP (adenosine triphosphate), which is a molecule that provides energy to cells and tissues. This increase in energy can help to improve nerve function and reduce the progression of neuropathy.

It is important to note that while infrared red light therapy has been shown to be effective in treating neuropathy in humans and pets, it should not be used as a substitute for conventional medical treatment and it is always recommended to consult a healthcare professional before starting any new form of therapy. Additionally, individual results may vary and multiple sessions may be needed for optimal results.

Skin conditions in humans and pets

Infrared red light therapy has been shown to be an effective treatment option for various skin conditions in humans and pets, including acne, eczema, psoriasis, and wrinkles.

The therapy works by penetrating the skin and tissues with low-level infrared light energy. This energy triggers a response in the cells and tissues, increasing their energy levels and boosting circulation. Improved circulation delivers oxygen and nutrients to the affected skin, promoting healing and reducing inflammation.

Infrared red light therapy has also been shown to stimulate the production of collagen, a key component of connective tissue, which can help to improve skin health and reduce the appearance of fine lines and wrinkles.

In addition to its anti-inflammatory effects, infrared red light therapy has also been shown to have an antimicrobial effect, which can help to reduce the severity of acne and other skin conditions caused by bacteria.

It is important to note that while infrared red light therapy has been shown to be effective in treating skin conditions in humans and pets, it should not be used as a substitute for conventional medical treatment and it is always recommended to consult a healthcare professional before starting any new form of therapy. Additionally, individual results may vary and multiple sessions may be needed for optimal results.

Wound healing in humans and pets

Infrared red light therapy has been shown to be an effective treatment option for wound healing in humans and pets. The therapy works by penetrating the skin and tissues with low-level infrared light energy, which triggers a response in the cells and tissues and boosts circulation.

Improved circulation delivers oxygen and nutrients to the affected area, promoting healing and reducing inflammation. Infrared red light therapy has also been shown to stimulate the production of ATP (adenosine triphosphate), a molecule that provides energy to cells and tissues, which can help to enhance the healing process.

In addition to its anti-inflammatory effects, infrared red light therapy has also been shown to have a positive effect on the production of collagen, a key component of connective tissue, which is important for wound healing. Increased collagen production can help to reduce the appearance of scars and improve the overall appearance of the affected area.

It is important to note that while infrared red light therapy has been shown to be effective in promoting wound healing in humans and pets, it should not be used as a substitute for conventional medical treatment and it is always recommended to consult a healthcare professional before starting any new form of therapy. Additionally, individual results may vary and multiple sessions may be needed for optimal results.

More research is being done...

Infrared red light therapy has been shown to be effective in treating a variety of other conditions in humans and pets, including:

1. **Muscle pain and soreness:** Infrared red light therapy can help to reduce pain and soreness in the muscles by increasing circulation and reducing inflammation.
2. **Tendonitis and bursitis:** Infrared red light therapy can help to reduce pain and inflammation in the tendons and bursae, promoting healing and reducing the risk of further injury.
3. **Chronic pain:** Infrared red light therapy has been shown to be effective in reducing chronic pain in the back, neck, and other areas of the body.
4. **Osteoarthritis:** Infrared red light therapy can help to reduce pain and inflammation in people with osteoarthritis, improving joint mobility and reducing the risk of further degeneration.
5. **Headaches and migraines:** Infrared red light therapy has been shown to help reduce the frequency and severity of headaches and migraines by reducing inflammation and increasing circulation to the head.
6. **Depression and anxiety:** Infrared red light therapy has been shown to have a positive effect on mood and can help to reduce symptoms of depression and anxiety by increasing the release of neurotransmitters in the brain.

Last but not least, we will talk about...

Non-traditional uses of Infrared Red Light Therapy.

While Infrared light therapy is primarily used for medical and therapeutic purposes, and as part of some spiritual practices, some people may incorporate infrared light therapy into their spiritual or religious practices, using it as a tool to promote healing and well-being on a spiritual level. Some proponents of spiritual or energy healing practices have suggested that the light energy can aid in clearing and aligning energy centers or chakras in the body, which is a concept in some Eastern spiritual practices.

It's important to note that these claims haven't been scientifically proven and traditional spiritual practices such as meditation, prayer and other rituals are still considered to be the main ways for people to access spiritual realms or powers. It's always a good idea to consult with a medical professional before starting any new therapy, including infrared light therapy, to be sure that it is appropriate and safe for your specific needs.

Can Infrared Red Light Therapy clear my chakras?

The concept of chakras, or energy centers in the body, is a central tenet of some Eastern spiritual practices, such as yoga and Ayurveda. According to this belief, when the chakras are balanced and aligned, the body and mind are in a state of harmony and well-being. It is suggested that when chakras are blocked, energy cannot flow freely, which can lead to physical, emotional or spiritual imbalance.

Some proponents of spiritual or energy healing practices have suggested that infrared light therapy can be used to clear and align the chakras by stimulating the flow of energy through the body. This is done by directing infrared light onto specific areas of the body, which correspond to the location of each chakra.

However, it's important to note that the claim that Infrared light therapy can clear and align chakras has not been scientifically proven. There are no studies or research that support this idea and its a concept that is not recognized by mainstream medicine or science. Also, it's important to keep in mind that the chakra system is not universally accepted in the field of psychology or spirituality.

While there may be some benefits to using infrared light therapy for physical and emotional well-being, it's important to consult with a medical professional before starting any new therapy, including infrared light therapy, to be sure that it is appropriate and safe for your specific needs.

It is important to note that while infrared red light therapy has been shown to be effective in treating these and other conditions, it should not be used as a substitute for conventional medical treatment and it is always recommended to consult a healthcare professional before starting any new form of therapy. Additionally, individual results may vary and multiple sessions may be needed for optimal results.

Why the Sacred Healing Infrared Light Therapy Belt is a great choice for beginners and experts

The Sacred Healing Infrared Light Therapy Belt is a versatile and effective tool for anyone looking to improve their health and well-being. Whether you are a beginner just starting to explore the benefits of infrared red light therapy or an experienced practitioner looking for a convenient and portable option, the Sacred Healing Infrared Light Therapy Belt offers something for everyone. With its advanced technology and easy-to-use design, this belt provides a simple and effective way to reap the many benefits of infrared red light therapy, from pain relief and improved circulation to accelerated healing and reduced inflammation. Whether you are dealing with a specific health condition or simply looking for a natural way to improve your overall health, the Sacred Healing Infrared Light Therapy Belt is a great choice for anyone looking to enhance their quality of life.

Advantages of using the Sacred Healing Infrared Light Therapy Belt

The Sacred Healing Infrared Light Therapy Belt offers several advantages to those looking to improve their health and well-being through infrared red light therapy:

1. **Convenience:** The belt design makes it easy to use, allowing you to apply infrared red light therapy directly to the affected area without having to disrobe or remove clothing.
2. **Portability:** The compact size of the Sacred Healing Infrared Light Therapy Belt makes it easy to take with you wherever you go, allowing you to enjoy the benefits of infrared red light therapy anytime, anywhere.
3. **Customization:** The Sacred Healing Infrared Light Therapy Belt allows you to adjust the intensity and duration of therapy to your specific needs, ensuring that you get the maximum benefits from each session.
4. **Effective:** The advanced technology used in the Sacred Healing Infrared Light Therapy Belt ensures that you receive optimal exposure to infrared red light, making it an effective way to improve your health and well-being.
5. **Safe:** Infrared red light therapy is a non-invasive, natural therapy that has been shown to be safe and effective for a wide range of health conditions. The Sacred Healing Infrared Light Therapy Belt uses only the highest quality components, ensuring that you receive safe, effective therapy.

These are just a few of the many advantages offered by the Sacred Healing Infrared Light Therapy Belt, making it a great choice for anyone looking to improve their health and well-being through infrared red light therapy.

Want more?

Other advantages of using the Sacred Healing Infrared Light Therapy Belt include:

1. **Ease of use:** The Sacred Healing Infrared Light Therapy Belt is simple and easy to use, even for those who are new to infrared red light therapy.
2. **Versatility:** The Sacred Healing Infrared Light Therapy Belt can be used to treat a wide range of health conditions, including pain, inflammation, skin conditions, and more.
3. **Time efficiency:** Infrared red light therapy sessions with the Sacred Healing Infrared Light Therapy Belt are typically short, making it a convenient and time-efficient way to improve your health.
4. **Cost-effectiveness:** Infrared red light therapy is a cost-effective alternative to traditional medical treatments, and the Sacred Healing Infrared Light Therapy Belt offers a convenient and affordable way to enjoy its benefits.
5. **Comfortable:** The Sacred Healing Infrared Light Therapy Belt is designed to be comfortable to wear, so you can relax and enjoy the therapy without feeling any discomfort.
6. **Durability:** The Sacred Healing Infrared Light Therapy Belt is built to last, so you can enjoy its benefits for years to come.
7. **Easy maintenance:** The Sacred Healing Infrared Light Therapy Belt is easy to clean and maintain, ensuring that you can use it as often as you like without any hassle.

Features of the Sacred Healing Infrared Light Therapy Belt

The Sacred Healing Infrared Light Therapy Belt is designed to provide an effective and convenient solution for individuals looking to improve their health and well-being. Here are some of its key features:

1. **Infrared light therapy:** The Sacred Healing Infrared Light Therapy Belt uses infrared red light therapy to penetrate deep into the skin, improving circulation, reducing pain and inflammation, and promoting healing.

2. **Adjustable fit:** The Sacred Healing Infrared Light Therapy Belt is designed to be adjustable, allowing you to achieve a comfortable and secure fit regardless of your body size and shape.

3. **Portable design:** The Sacred Healing Infrared Light Therapy Belt is designed to be portable, so you can enjoy its benefits at home, at work, or on-the-go.

4. **Easy control:** The Sacred Healing Infrared Light Therapy Belt is equipped with simple and intuitive controls, making it easy for you to adjust the therapy to your preferences.

5. **Durable materials:** The Sacred Healing Infrared Light Therapy Belt is made of high-quality materials that are built to last, ensuring that you can enjoy its benefits for years to come.

6. **Safe and non-invasive:** The Sacred Healing Infrared Light Therapy Belt is a safe and non-invasive solution for those looking to improve their health and well-being.

7. **Multi-functional:** The Sacred Healing Infrared Light Therapy Belt is designed to be multi-functional, allowing you to treat a wide range of health conditions with ease.

8. **Convenient storage:** The Sacred Healing Infrared Light Therapy Belt comes with a convenient storage case, making it easy to transport and store when not in use.

How the Sacred Healing Infrared Light Therapy Belt compares to other infrared light therapy devices

The Sacred Healing Infrared Light Therapy Belt compares favorably to other infrared light therapy devices in several ways:

1. **Convenience:** The Sacred Healing Infrared Light Therapy Belt is designed to be portable and can be used at home, at work, or on-the-go, whereas some other infrared light therapy devices are stationary and can only be used in one location.
2. **Adjustable fit:** The Sacred Healing Infrared Light Therapy Belt is designed to be adjustable, allowing you to achieve a comfortable and secure fit regardless of your body size and shape. Other infrared light therapy devices may not be as adjustable, making it difficult to achieve the desired fit.
3. **Easy control:** The Sacred Healing Infrared Light Therapy Belt is equipped with simple and intuitive controls, making it easy for you to adjust the therapy to your preferences. Some other infrared light therapy devices may have complicated or confusing controls.
4. **Durable materials:** The Sacred Healing Infrared Light Therapy Belt is made of high-quality materials that are built to last, ensuring that you can enjoy its benefits for years to come. Some other infrared light therapy devices may be made of lower-quality materials that are more prone to wear and tear.

5. **Versatility:** The Sacred Healing Infrared Light Therapy Belt is designed to be multi-functional, allowing you to treat a wide range of health conditions with ease. Some other infrared light therapy devices may only be able to treat a limited range of conditions.

6. **Affordability:** The Sacred Healing Infrared Light Therapy Belt offers a cost-effective solution for individuals looking to improve their health and well-being, making it a great choice for both beginners and experts. Some other infrared light therapy devices may be more expensive and not as accessible to a wider range of individuals.

Why the Sacred Healing Infrared Light Therapy Belt is the perfect starting point for learning about infrared light therapy

The Sacred Healing Infrared Light Therapy Belt offers a great starting point for those who are interested in learning about the benefits of infrared light therapy. This device is designed to be user-friendly and easy to use, making it accessible to individuals of all experience levels. The compact size and adjustable strap of the belt make it a convenient option for use at home or on-the-go. Furthermore, its high-quality components and advanced technology provide powerful and effective infrared therapy, delivering the same benefits as larger and more expensive devices. With its affordable price point, the Sacred Healing Infrared Light Therapy Belt is a great investment for those looking to explore the world of infrared therapy and improve their overall health and well-being.

Safety and Side Effects of Infrared Red Light Therapy

Infrared red light therapy is generally considered to be a safe and non-invasive form of therapy. However, as with any form of therapy, it is important to be aware of the potential side effects and risks associated with its use. In this chapter, we will discuss the safety and side effects of infrared red light therapy, and provide information on how to minimize the risk of adverse effects. By understanding the safety and side effects of infrared therapy, you can make an informed decision on whether this form of therapy is right for you and your needs.

Is Infrared Red Light Therapy Safe for humans and pets?

Infrared red light therapy is generally considered safe for humans and pets. The therapy uses low-level, non-ionizing infrared light to penetrate deep into the skin, which has been shown to be safe for human and animal use. Infrared light therapy is a non-invasive, painless procedure that does not involve any surgical procedures or the use of drugs, making it a popular choice for those seeking a natural and safe form of therapy.

Additionally, the low-level of infrared light used in therapy is not strong enough to cause any harm to cells, tissues, or DNA, making it a safe option for use on all parts of the body. The therapy has been widely used for several decades and has a proven track record of being safe and effective for the treatment of various conditions.

However, it is important to note that as with any form of therapy, some individuals may experience side effects or skin irritation. It is recommended to consult with a healthcare professional prior to using infrared light therapy, particularly if you have any underlying medical conditions or are pregnant. Furthermore, individuals with skin conditions such as eczema or sensitive skin should also consult with a healthcare professional before using infrared light therapy.

In conclusion, when used properly and under the guidance of a healthcare professional, infrared red light therapy is considered safe for both humans and pets.

Potential side effects for humans and pets

Infrared red light therapy is generally considered safe for humans and pets, with minimal side effects reported. However, it is important to be aware of the potential risks and to follow recommended guidelines for usage. In some cases, people may experience skin irritation, eye strain or sensitivity, or headaches after exposure to the light therapy. Additionally, individuals with certain medical conditions, such as lupus or cataracts, may be advised against using the therapy. For pets, there is a potential for skin irritation or sensitivity, particularly if they have pre-existing skin conditions. It is important to speak with a veterinarian before using infrared red light therapy on your pet to ensure it is safe and appropriate for their individual needs. Overall, it is essential to follow recommended guidelines for usage and to consult with a doctor or veterinarian before starting the therapy, especially if you have a pre-existing medical condition.

Contraindications for humans and pets

Infrared red light therapy is not recommended or contraindicated for certain individuals and conditions. For humans, it is important to speak with a doctor before undergoing the therapy if you have a pre-existing medical condition, such as lupus, cataracts, or any type of light sensitivity. Additionally, individuals who have had recent eye surgery, have a history of seizures, or are pregnant should avoid the therapy.

For pets, it is also important to consult with a veterinarian before starting the therapy, particularly if your pet has a pre-existing medical condition, such as eye disease or skin sensitivity. Additionally, pets who have had recent eye surgery or have a history of light sensitivity should avoid the therapy. It is important to follow recommended guidelines for usage and to only use infrared red light therapy under the guidance of a healthcare professional to ensure the safety and well-being of both humans and pets.

Choosing the Right Infrared Red Light Therapy Device

Infrared red light therapy is a non-invasive and natural approach to healing and wellness. With its numerous benefits and growing popularity, it's no wonder that the market is now filled with a wide range of infrared red light therapy devices. From handheld devices to full-body light therapy systems, the choices can be overwhelming. That's why it's important to understand the key factors to consider when choosing the right infrared red light therapy device for you or your pet.

Factors to consider when choosing an Infrared Light Therapy device for humans and pets

When choosing an infrared red light therapy device, there are several factors to consider, including:

1. **Wavelength:** Different wavelengths are effective for different conditions, so it's important to choose a device with the right wavelength for your specific needs.
2. **Power:** Infrared light therapy devices can vary in power, which is measured in milliwatts (mW). Higher power devices are often more effective, but also more expensive.

3. **Size:** Consider the size of the device, as larger devices may be more cumbersome to use, while smaller devices may not cover enough surface area for your needs.

4. **Portability:** Some devices are portable and can be used anywhere, while others are stationary and require a power source.

5. **Cost:** Infrared light therapy devices can range in cost from under $100 to several thousand dollars. Consider your budget and the value you're getting for your money.

6. **Safety features:** Some devices have safety features such as built-in timers and automatic shut-off to ensure safe use.

7. **Customer reviews:** Read customer reviews to get a better understanding of the experiences others have had with the device you're considering.

It's also important to consult with a healthcare professional, especially if you have a pre-existing medical condition or are taking any medications, to ensure that infrared light therapy is safe and appropriate for you. The same goes for pets, a veterinary professional should be consulted before using infrared light therapy.

Types of Infrared Light Therapy devices for humans and pets

There are several types of Infrared Light Therapy devices available for humans and pets. The most common types are:

1. **Infrared Light Therapy Lamps and Panels:** These are stationary devices that emit red and near-infrared light to penetrate the skin and tissues.

2. **Infrared Light Therapy Wraps:** These are devices that are worn around specific parts of the body and

emit red and near-infrared light to help treat pain, inflammation, and promote healing.

3. **Infrared Light Therapy Gloves and Socks:** These are devices designed for hands and feet and emit red and near-infrared light to help improve circulation, reduce pain and swelling, and promote healing.

4. **Infrared Light Therapy Belts:** These are devices designed for the waist and emit red and near-infrared light to help reduce pain, improve circulation, and promote healing in the lower back, hips, and legs.

5. **Infrared Light Therapy Pads:** These are devices designed for use on a flat surface and emit red and near-infrared light to help treat pain, inflammation, and promote healing in various parts of the body.

It's important to choose an Infrared Light Therapy device that is appropriate for your specific needs, as well as one that is of good quality and from a reputable manufacturer.

How to use Infrared Light Therapy devices for humans and pets

Infrared light therapy devices can be used by humans and pets in a variety of ways. For humans, the most common method is to use handheld devices or panels that can be directed towards the affected area of the body. In pets, devices can be used directly on the skin or placed near them to allow for indirect exposure. It is important to follow the manufacturer's instructions for use, including the recommended time for each session and the proper distance to maintain between the device and the skin. Additionally, it is recommended to start with shorter sessions and gradually increase the time as tolerated to minimize any potential discomfort. To achieve optimal results, it is best to use infrared light therapy devices regularly and consistently.

Conclusion

In the conclusion chapter, it is time to summarize the key takeaways and highlights of the information discussed throughout the book about Infrared Red Light Therapy. This chapter will reflect on the benefits and advantages of this form of therapy and the reasons why it is becoming a popular choice for individuals seeking non-invasive, natural and effective solutions for various health and wellness needs. The purpose of this chapter is to provide readers with a clear understanding of how Infrared Red Light Therapy works and how it can help enhance their quality of life, whether for themselves or their beloved pets.

Summary of the benefits of Infrared Red Light Therapy for humans and pets

Infrared red light therapy has been shown to have a range of benefits for both humans and pets. It is a non-invasive and safe form of therapy that utilizes the therapeutic properties of red and near-infrared light to promote healing and provide pain relief. This therapy has been found to be effective in treating a range of conditions, including arthritis, joint pain, neuropathy, skin conditions, and wound healing. It can also help improve circulation, reduce inflammation, boost immunity, and reduce stress and anxiety.

Infrared light therapy works by penetrating deep into the skin and stimulating cellular activity. This increased activity can help speed up the healing process, improve circulation, and reduce inflammation. Infrared light therapy is also believed to promote the production of ATP (adenosine triphosphate), which is the energy currency of the cell. This increased energy can help cells repair and regenerate more efficiently, leading to improved overall health.

In conclusion, Infrared red light therapy is a safe and effective form of therapy for humans and pets that has been shown to provide a range of benefits. Whether you are suffering from a specific condition or simply looking to improve your overall health and wellness, this form of therapy may be the solution you have been looking for. With a wide range of devices available, it is important to choose the right one for your needs and to use it as directed for the best results.

Final thoughts on Infrared Red Light Therapy as an alternative to traditional treatments for humans and pets

As I come to the end of this journey through the world of Infrared Red Light Therapy, I am filled with a sense of wonder and gratitude. From the research and experiences shared, it is evident that Infrared Red Light Therapy is a powerful alternative to traditional treatments for humans and pets. Its benefits range from reducing pain and inflammation, improving circulation, promoting healing and skin health, to treating a variety of conditions, and even reducing stress and anxiety.

What I find truly remarkable about Infrared Red Light Therapy is its non-invasive nature, making it a safe and gentle option for those who seek natural remedies. Furthermore, the advancements in technology have made it possible for individuals to access infrared light therapy devices, such as the Sacred Healing Infrared Light Therapy Belt, from the comfort of their own homes.

As an award-winning author, it gives me great satisfaction to see how this alternative form of therapy has changed the lives of so many people and their pets. It is a privilege to have had the opportunity to share this knowledge with the world, and I hope that this book will inspire more individuals to explore the potential of Infrared Red Light Therapy as a tool for improving their health and well-being.

In conclusion, Infrared Red Light Therapy is a fascinating and innovative alternative to traditional treatments. It has the potential to revolutionize the way we approach our health, offering a safe and natural solution for a range of physical and mental conditions. I am confident that as more research is conducted, we will continue to uncover the endless possibilities of this incredible therapy.

"The Sacred Healing Light: Unlocking the Power of Infrared Red Light Therapy for Humans and Pets"

Written By Michael DiCicco & Estrella Ortega
Edited by Al Indira

About The Authors

Michael DiCicco is a seasoned entrepreneur and expert in the field of infrared technology. With over two decades of experience in the industry, he is a former Vice President of Infrared Sciences at Computer Vision Systems Laboratories (CVSL), a publicly traded company. Throughout his career, he has been a pioneer in the development and implementation of cutting-edge infrared technology for a variety of applications. Today, he co-owns Sacred Healing Supply Company, a company dedicated to bringing the benefits of infrared light therapy to people and pets everywhere. With his extensive knowledge and passion for infrared light therapy, Michael is dedicated to helping people lead healthier, more vibrant lives.

Estrella Ortega is a renowned alternative medicine practitioner and the co-owner of Sacred Healing Supply Company. She has been passionate about natural and holistic healing methods for over a decade, and has dedicated her life to helping people find relief from pain, stress and other conditions through the use of innovative and cutting-edge products such as infrared light therapy. With her extensive knowledge and experience in the field, Estrella has become a trusted expert in the alternative medicine community and is committed to providing her clients with the best possible care and results. Whether through her products or her one-on-one consultations, Estrella is dedicated to helping her clients achieve optimal health and wellness.

Michael DiCicco and Estrella Ortega shared a common passion for alternative healing methods and a desire to help those in need. They combined their expertise in infrared technology and alternative medicine to form Sacred Healing Supply Company. Starting from a small, home-based operation, they worked tirelessly to provide high-quality infrared products and educate people on the benefits of infrared therapy. With their dedication and commitment, they have grown Sacred Healing Supply Company into a trusted and well-respected provider of infrared therapy products, making a positive impact on the lives of countless people and pets.

About Sacred Healing
Supply Company

"Honoring tradition, embracing innovation" -
Sacred Healing Supply Company

At Sacred Healing Supply Company, we believe that technology and ancient wisdom can work together to promote healing and well-being. Our mission is to provide individuals with the latest in cutting-edge technology and traditional spiritual tools and resources. We strive to empower people to take an active role in their own healing journey by offering a wide range of products and services that integrate technology and spiritual practices. Our goal is to create a sense of balance and harmony in people's lives by combining the best of both worlds and helping people access the power of the sacred and the benefits of technology to promote physical, emotional, and spiritual well-being.